Best Sex Positions to Help You Last Longer in Bed

20+ Expert-Approved Positions That'll Make Sex Last Longer plus Top Sex Tips for Premature Ejaculation

Cheryl Bach

Best Sex Positions to Help You Last Longer in Bed

Publisher: IntimateInk Press

Email: intimateinkpress@gmail.com

Cover design by IntimateInk Press

Interior layout and design by IntimateInk Press

Printed in USA

Fonts: Google fonts

Image: Freepik.com. This cover has been designed using assets from Freepik.com

For permission to use copyrighted material from this book, please contact the copyright holder listed above.

First Edition: 2024

Distributed by Amazon.com, Inc.

Cheryl Bach

Table of Contents

Cheryl Bach

Chapter 1

Introduction

Sex is an essential part of life, and for many people, it's a source of pleasure, intimacy, and connection with their partners. However, experiencing premature ejaculation can put a damper on these benefits. In this book, we will explore the link between sex positions and lasting longer in bed.

Why it's important to address Premature Ejaculation (PE)

Premature ejaculation happens when a man ejaculates before they want to or shortly after penetration. It's a common occurrence, affecting up to 1 in 3 men, yet it remains one of the most challenging sexual problems to

Best Sex Positions to Help You Last Longer in Bed

address. Untreated, PE can lead to stress, anxiety, and depression. It can also negatively impact men's self-esteem and their relationship with their partner. That's why learning techniques to address PE is crucial to improve sexual performance, boost confidence, and foster a stronger connection with our partners.

The Link between Sex Positions and Lasting Longer

Sex positions are not just about finding a comfortable angle or hitting that one sweet spot. In fact, certain sex positions can help you take control of your sexual response, enabling you to prevent premature ejaculation and prolong your sexual experience. We will discuss how different positions can impact your stimulation and explore which ones are beneficial for lasting longer in bed.

Cheryl Bach

The Benefits of Using Different Positions in Bed

Using different sex positions offer various benefits beyond lasting longer in bed. These advantages include adding variety and excitement to your sexual repertoire, intensifying orgasms, increasing intimacy, and strengthening the romantic bond with your partner. By exploring a wide range of positions, you can break out of the monotony of your sex life, improve communication with your partner, and discover new ways to experience pleasure.

In conclusion, the introduction will set the tone for this book, highlighting the importance of addressing premature ejaculation, exploring the link between sex positions and lasting longer, and the benefits of using different positions in bed. This book will provide you with practical tips, techniques, and expert-approved sex positions to help you take control of your sexual response, improve your performance, and enhance your sexual relationship with your partner.

Cheryl Bach

Chapter 2

Missionary Variations

Traditional Missionary Position and Why It's a Great Starting Point

The traditional missionary position is one of the most popular and widely used sex positions globally. It involves lying flat on your back, while your partner is on top, with their legs between yours. While this position is simple and straightforward, it provides maximum intimacy, full body contact, and an opportunity for deep emotional connection.

Cheryl Bach

Modifications to the Classic Position That Can Help You Last Longer

While the classic missionary position can be fantastic for intimacy and pleasure, certain modifications can help those who struggle with premature ejaculation. One such modification involves propping your pelvis with a pillow or two to improve the angle of penetration and reduce the amount of friction from your partner's vaginal muscles, which can cause overstimulation.

Another modification involves controlling the pace of thrusting by using your hands or forearms to hold your partner's hips and regulate the speed. Slowing down the pace can help prolong the sexual experience, increase intimacy, and enhance the orgasms for both partners.

Tips for Communication and Making Adjustments with Your Partner

Communication is an essential part of any sexual relationship, and it's crucial to discuss modifications or adjustments to the missionary position that can benefit both partners. The key is to approach the conversation openly, honestly, and without judgment. Both partners should feel comfortable giving feedback and suggestions to improve the experience. It's essential to understand that sexual pleasure is a journey and not a destination; it requires patience, exploration, and experimentation to find what works best for you both.

In conclusion, missionary variations provide an excellent starting point for exploring different sex positions and techniques to improve sexual performance, increase intimacy, and enhance the orgasms for both partners. Modifications such as pelvic propping and pace control can help those dealing with premature ejaculation to last longer in bed and prolong the sexual experience. Effective communication between partners is critical to making adjustments that benefit both partners. By utilizing these tips in your sexual repertoire, you and your partner can enhance your sexual relationship and enjoy a more fulfilling and satisfying experience.

Chapter 3

Cowgirl and Reverse Cowgirl

Cowgirl and reverse cowgirl are two of the most popular sex positions, and for good reason. These positions offer a range of benefits that can help you to last longer in bed, increase intimacy and pleasure, and intensify orgasms.

Overview of Cowgirl and Reverse Cowgirl Positions

The cowgirl position involves the partner taking the dominant position by straddling their partner while facing them, either sitting up or leaning forward. In contrast, the reverse cowgirl position is the same but with one major difference: the partner faces away from the person they are straddling.

Cheryl Bach

These positions offer several benefits, including direct clitoral stimulation, increased control for the receiving partner, deep penetration, and visual appeal. But what many people don't know is that these positions also enable you to take control of your orgasm and last longer in bed.

Techniques for Slowing Down and Taking Control

Both cowgirl and reverse cowgirl positions are great for slowing down and taking control over your sexual response. By using certain techniques, you can build up your stamina and help yourself to last longer in bed.

One effective technique is to use a circular grinding motion during penetration, rather than the traditional up-and-down bouncing movement. This motion reduces the level of friction and provides a more controlled pace that can help you last longer. It also allows for increased clitoral stimulation and a higher level of intimacy and connection between partners.

Another technique is to use deep, slow breathing to relax your body and reduce tension in your muscles. As you feel yourself nearing orgasm, take a deep inhale through your nose and slowly exhale through your mouth. This will help to regulate your breathing and maintain a sense of calm and control. You can also adjust the angle of penetration to reduce sensitivity and prolong the experience. By leaning forward or backward, you can change the depth and angle of penetration, which can reduce pressure on the sensitive areas of the penis and help you last longer.

How to Communicate Effectively and Make Adjustments to Suit Both Partners

As with any sexual position or technique, communication is key to ensuring mutual pleasure and satisfaction. It's essential to communicate openly and honestly with your partner, expressing your likes and dislikes while also listening to their preferences. Every individual is different, and what works for one person may not work for another, so it's important to make adjustments that suit both partners.

One effective way to communicate is to use nonverbal cues, such as pulling back or pausing during penetration, which can signal to your partner that you need a break or are approaching orgasm. This allows them to slow down or change their pace, providing you with the opportunity to regain control and prolong the experience.

Another effective strategy is to try different variations of the cowgirl and reverse cowgirl positions, such as incorporating a sex toy or using a prop like a pillow to adjust the angle of penetration. These modifications can help to reduce sensitivity and increase stimulation, providing new sensations and experiences for both partners.

In conclusion, the cowgirl and reverse cowgirl positions offer a wealth of benefits for couples looking to last longer

Best Sex Positions to Help You Last Longer in Bed

in bed and explore new levels of intimacy and pleasure. By using techniques like circular grinding and deep breathing, and communicating effectively with your partner, you can take control over your body and experience more satisfying and pleasurable sexual encounters.

21

Chapter 4

Doggy Style Variations

Doggy style is one of the most popular and versatile sex positions, offering a range of advantages that can help you to last longer in bed, enhance intimacy, and increase the intensity of orgasm. In this chapter, we'll explore the variations of this classic position and provide tips for pacing yourself and incorporating manual stimulation.

Explanation of the Doggy Style Position and Its Variations

The doggy style position involves one partner penetrating the other from behind while on all fours. This position is great for deep penetration, G-spot stimulation, and visual appeal. Additionally, it can be modified to suit a range of preferences and physical abilities.

Some popular variations of doggy style include:

Standing doggy style: This variation involves one partner standing while the other is on all fours. The standing partner can use the wall or furniture for support while thrusting.

Sloppy doggy style: This variation involves the penetrating partner tilting slightly to one side, allowing for better access to the G-spot and a tighter fit.

Scratching doggy style: In this variation, the receiver scratches their own back while the penetrating partner watches or scratches along with them.

Perfect doggy style: This variation involves the penetrating partner staying very still, while the receiving partner does most of the work by gyrating their hips in a grinding motion.

These variations can provide new sensations and experiences while still utilizing the benefits of deep penetration and visual appeal.

Techniques for Pacing and Slowing Down to Last Longer

One of the biggest benefits of doggy style is the level of control that it offers. By using certain techniques, you can slow down and pace yourself, increasing your stamina and helping you to last longer.

Here are some effective techniques to try:

Use shallow strokes: Rather than thrusting deeply and quickly, try using shallow strokes that focus on the opening of the vagina or anus. This reduces the level of stimulation and allows you to maintain control for longer.

Use a grind rather than thrusting: Instead of thrusting in and out, try a circular grinding motion, which can provide a lower level of friction and reduce sensitivity.

Pause when nearing orgasm: If you feel yourself nearing orgasm, take a break for a few seconds before continuing. This can help you to regain control and prolong the experience.

Change positions or adjust angles: Changing the angle of penetration or switching to a different position can help to reduce sensitivity and prolong the experience.

How to Incorporate Manual Stimulation for Both Yourself and Your Partner

Manual stimulation can be a great addition to doggy style, enhancing pleasure and intimacy for both partners.

Here are some tips for incorporating manual stimulation into your sex life:

Use your hands: While penetrating from behind, use one hand to stimulate yourself or your partner's clitoris or penis. This provides an extra level of stimulation while also reducing sensitivity.

Try adding a vibrator: Adding a vibrator to the mix can increase sensations and provide new experiences for both partners.

Experiment with rimming: Rimming, or using the tongue to stimulate the anus, can provide intense pleasure and enhance intimacy during doggy style.

When incorporating manual stimulation, it's important to communicate with your partner and be mindful of their preferences and boundaries. Experiment with different techniques and find what works best for you and your partner.

In conclusion, doggy style is a versatile and popular sex position with a range of variations that can provide new sensations and experiences. By using techniques like shallow strokes and changing angles, and incorporating manual stimulation, you can take control over your body and increase intimacy and pleasure with your partner. Remember to communicate effectively and experiment with different techniques to find what works best for you and your partner. Enjoy!

Chapter 5

Spooning Positions

Spooning positions are an excellent way to enjoy intimate, connected sex while also promoting a sense of closeness. In this chapter, we'll explore some of the best spooning positions and provide techniques for controlling your breathing and pacing for longer sex.

Overview of Spooning Positions

Spooning positions are named due to the way in which one partner "spoons" the other, with their bodies positioned close together.

Here are some popular spooning positions:

The Lazy Spoon: One partner lies on their side facing away from the other, while the second partner spoons them from behind. This position allows for deep penetration and can be adjusted to suit each partner's comfort level.

The Big Spoon Position: This position is similar to the lazy spoon, but the penetrating partner is the "big spoon". This position offers a greater sense of control and allows for close body contact.

The Snuggle Spoon: In this position, both partners lie on their sides facing each other, with the penetrating partner behind the receiving partner. This position offers a greater sense of intimacy and allows for more physical touch.

Techniques for Controlling Your Breathing and Pacing to Last Longer

Spooning positions are ideal for those looking to last longer during sex, as they offer a level of control and comfort that is hard to match.

Here are some techniques you can use to control your breathing and pacing during spooning:

Take deep breaths: Focused, deep breathing can help to reduce anxiety and tension, controlling your pace and allowing you to last longer.

Try the start-stop technique: This involves pausing during sex when you feel yourself nearing orgasm to slow down and calm your breathing. Resume when you feel ready to continue, and repeat as necessary.

Cheryl Bach

Change the pace: Varying the pace of your thrusts can help you to last longer by reducing stimulation and increasing control.

Tips for Incorporating Intimacy and Connection in These Positions

Spooning positions are a natural way to incorporate intimacy and connection into your sex life.

Here are some tips for taking advantage of these benefits:

Use eye contact: Looking into your partner's eyes during spooning can increase intimacy and emotional connection.

Hold each other close: Wrapping your arms around each other can provide a sense of safety and create a deeper bond between partners.

Best Sex Positions to Help You Last Longer in Bed

Focus on touch: Sensual touching, massaging, and kissing can provide physical pleasure while also building emotional intimacy.

In conclusion, spooning positions offer a fantastic way to promote intimacy and connected sex while providing exceptional control to help you last longer in bed. Experiment with different spooning positions like the lazy spoon, big spoon position, and snuggle spoon and remember to incorporate focused breathing techniques to maintain control and last longer. Finally, don't forget to prioritize physical touch, eye contact, and emotional closeness to enjoy an unforgettable, intimate experience with your partner.

Chapter 6

Standing and Other Unique Positions

In this chapter, we'll explore standing positions, like standing doggy style and the standing missionary position, as well as some other unique positions that can help extend sex and prevent premature ejaculation. Modifications for these positions to suit individual needs and preferences will be also discussed.

Explanation of Standing Positions

Standing positions can add a level of intensity and novelty to sexual encounters while also facilitating deeper penetration and increasing sensations.

Cheryl Bach

Here are some popular standing positions:

Standing Doggy Style: In this position, one partner stands and leans forward, while the other penetrates from behind. This position offers deep penetration and intense stimulation, but it can also cause fatigue in the penetrating partner.

Standing Missionary Position: This variation of the missionary position involves one partner standing against a wall or sturdy surface with their legs spread apart, while the other penetrates while standing. This position allows for a deep connection with eye contact while still maintaining the benefits of standing positions.

Tips for Using Other Unique Positions to Prevent Premature Ejaculation

There are many unique positions that can be used to prevent premature ejaculation and prolong sexual encounters.

Here are some tips for incorporating them into your sex life:

The Coital Alignment Technique (CAT): This technique involves aligning the pubic bone with the clitoris to promote clitoral stimulation via grinding and hip motion. This technique reduces intense stimulation and allows for increased control, leading to longer-lasting sex.

Reverse Cowgirl: In this position, the penetrating partner lies on their back while the receiving partner straddles them facing away. This position allows for greater control over depth and speed, as well as some clitoral stimulation depending on the angle.

The Lotus: This position involves seated partners, with the penetrating partner sitting cross-legged while the receiving partner straddles them, wrapping their legs around the penetrating partner's waist. This position is great for a deeper connection and can allow for greater control over timing and pace.

Modifications for These Positions to Suit Individual Needs and Preferences

Every individual has unique preferences and needs in terms of sexual positions, so it's important to modify these positions to enhance their experience.

Here are some modifications for standing and unique positions:

Use a Wall or Surface: Incorporating a wall or sturdy surface can provide support for the standing partner, increasing comfort and control.

Adjust Depth and Angle: Varying depth and angle of penetration can provide increased control and pacing.

Experiment with Lighting and Environment: Dimming the lights or trying different environments can enhance the experience and provide a more intimate setting.

Add Toys and Lubricants: Adding sex toys or lubricants can increase stimulation while also reducing friction and providing smoother movements.

Communicate with Your Partner: Communication is key in any sexual encounter, so it's important to discuss preferences, needs, and comfort levels throughout the experience.

In conclusion, standing positions offer a unique and intense sexual experience, while other unique positions like the Coital Alignment Technique, Reverse Cowgirl, and The Lotus can provide greater control and pacing. Modifying these positions to suit individual needs and preferences is key to a fulfilling and successful sexual encounter.

Cheryl Bach

Remember to communicate, experiment, and prioritize intimacy and connection for an unforgettable experience.

Chapter 7

Sex Tips for Premature Ejaculation

Premature ejaculation can be a frustrating and embarrassing issue for many men, but there are ways to overcome it and enjoy longer and more satisfying sexual encounters. In this chapter, we'll explore additional tips and techniques for lasting longer in bed, the importance of relaxation, mindfulness, and breathing exercises, and ways to increase stamina for longer sex sessions.

Additional Tips and Techniques for Lasting Longer in Bed

There are many tips and techniques that can help you last longer in bed and prevent premature ejaculation. Here are some expert-approved options:

Kegel Exercises: Kegel exercises focus on strengthening the pelvic muscles that control ejaculation. These exercises can be done anywhere and can greatly improve sexual stamina over time.

The "Start-Stop" Method: This method involves reaching the brink of ejaculation and then stopping all sexual activity until the urge to ejaculate subsides. This technique is repeated several times during sexual activity and can help you gain greater control over your ejaculation.

The "Squeeze" Technique: This technique involves pressing on the base of the penis when you feel close to ejaculation, reducing stimulation and delaying ejaculation. Similar to the "Start-Stop" method, this technique can be practiced repeatedly.

Best Sex Positions to Help You Last Longer in Bed

Using a Condom: Wearing a condom during sexual activity can reduce sensitivity and provide an extra layer of physical protection that can help prolong sexual encounters.

The Importance of Relaxation, Mindfulness, and Breathing Exercises

Premature ejaculation can often stem from anxiety, stress, and other psychological factors. Incorporating relaxation, mindfulness, and breathing exercises can help alleviate these issues and improve sexual performance.

Here are some techniques for relaxation, mindfulness, and breathing exercises:

Deep Breathing: Deep breathing exercises can help you relax and reduce stress and anxiety. Take slow, deep breaths in through your nose and then exhale slowly through your mouth.

Muscle Relaxation: Relaxing your muscles can reduce tension and increase relaxation. Focus on tensing each muscle group in your body, and then release the tension slowly.

Visualization: Visualization techniques involve imagining a calming and relaxing environment or scene. Visualize yourself in a peaceful place and focus on the sensory details of your surroundings.

Mindfulness Meditation: Mindfulness meditation involves focusing on the present moment without judgment or distraction. This can help reduce stress and anxiety and improve overall relaxation.

Ways to Increase Stamina for Longer Sex Sessions

Increasing stamina is an important aspect of lasting longer in bed and preventing premature ejaculation.

Best Sex Positions to Help You Last Longer in Bed

Here are some ways to increase your sexual stamina:

Exercise: Regular exercise can improve cardiovascular health and increase overall endurance, which can provide a significant boost to sexual stamina.

Healthy Diet: A healthy diet can provide the necessary nutrients and energy for sexual activity and overall wellbeing. Avoiding foods that are high in sugar and fat can also help improve stamina.

Communication with Partner: Communication with your sexual partner is crucial in helping to last longer in bed. Discussing preferences, needs, and limitations can help both partners feel more comfortable and satisfied during sexual activity.

Cheryl Bach

Masturbation Exercises: Practicing masturbation exercises, such as the "Stop-Start" technique or the "Squeeze" technique, can help improve control over ejaculation and increase sexual stamina.

In conclusion, premature ejaculation can be a frustrating issue for many men, but there are techniques and tips that can help increase sexual stamina and prevent premature ejaculation. Incorporating relaxation, mindfulness, and breathing exercises and actively working on strengthening pelvic muscles can contribute to better control over ejaculation. Discussing desires, preferences and limitations with your partner and practicing masturbation exercises can also help men last longer in bed. Additionally, maintaining a healthy diet with regular exercise can lead to improved cardiovascular health and overall endurance, which can contribute to longer and more satisfying sexual encounters. With practice and patience, premature ejaculation can be a thing of the past.

Chapter 8

Conclusion

In this book, we've explored numerous ways to help improve sexual stamina, delay ejaculation and achieve longer and more satisfying sexual encounters. We've discussed expert-approved sex positions, techniques for lasting longer in bed, tips for managing premature ejaculation, and ways to incorporate relaxation and breathing exercises.

Using different sex positions can certainly contribute to better control over your ejaculation and to increase overall sexual pleasure for both partners. Finding the right position(s) for you and your partner could take some experimentation, but it's worth the effort for the hugely beneficial results obtained from slow, sensual, and intimate sex experience.

It's important to remember that communication is key when it comes to sexual experiences. Sharing likes, dislikes, and open communication will improve trust, intimacy, and overall satisfaction in the encounter. This will ensure a pleasurable experience for both partners and enhance the emotional bond between you and your partner. It's essential to be honest and open about your needs, desires, and boundaries, so both of you can feel more comfortable exploring new positions and techniques together.

Instead of feeling ashamed or embarrassed about premature ejaculation, use it as an opportunity to try new things with your partner and explore various techniques that can help improve your sexual stamina.

It's worth noting that trying out different sexual positions alone may not solve the whole problem if the underlying issue is related to anxiety, stress, or other psychological factors. Therefore, incorporating relaxation techniques such as breathing exercises, meditation and mindfulness can help address these causes.

Remember, lasting longer in bed takes practice, patience, and an open mind. Don't be afraid to experiment with new techniques, and always prioritize communication with your partner, honesty, and respect for each other's needs. With time and effort, you and your partner can experience longer and more satisfying sexual encounters that strengthen your emotional bond and overall relationship.

In conclusion, the importance of sexual pleasure and satisfaction cannot be overemphasized in relationships. Premature ejaculation or lack of control over ejaculation is a common problem among men, but it shouldn't limit the potential for intimacy and satisfying sex life. Experimenting with different sex positions, incorporating relaxation techniques, using various techniques to improve stamina, and involving communication between you and your partner can all help to achieve longer and more enjoyable sexual experiences for both partners.

It's important to remember that everyone's body is different, and what works for one person may not work for another. The key is to find what helps you and your partner enjoy sex the most, and to approach it with an open mind and willingness to learn and grow together. With the information book, we hope you feel more confident and equipped to overcome premature ejaculation and improve your overall sexual health and wellbeing.

Don't forget that sex is supposed to be fun and enjoyable! So, try not to get too caught up in the technical aspects of lasting longer in bed. Instead, focus on the pleasure and

Best Sex Positions to Help You Last Longer in Bed

connection between you and your partner, and enjoy the moment.

We hope this book has been helpful in providing valuable information and advice on sex positions and techniques that can help you last longer in bed. Remember that improving your sexual stamina is a journey, and it's up to you and your partner to work together towards building long-lasting and satisfying sexual experiences.

Now that you have a plethora of information to guide you, it's time to start exploring and having fun with your partner. Good luck and happy exploring!